RBT Exam Prep 2024-2025

Lisa Stiffler

RBT EXAM GUIDE

OVERVIEW

The RBT exam stands as a pivotal evaluation mechanism, uniquely tailored to scrutinize the depth of knowledge, practical aptitude, and ethical acumen of aspiring Registered Behavior Technicians (RBTs). This examination serves as an indispensable cornerstone within the certification process, meticulously crafted to ensure that RBTs possess the requisite proficiencies essential for delivering ABA therapy of the highest caliber.

Understanding the RBT exam entails delving into the intricate landscape of a profession dedicated to providing crucial support in the realm of behavioral therapy. Registered Behavior Technicians (RBTs) serve as pivotal figures in the realm of Applied Behavior Analysis (ABA) therapy, leveraging their expertise to facilitate positive change in individuals' lives.

At the helm of this profession are the Board Certified Behavior Analysts (BCBAs), who oversee and guide the work of RBTs. While BCBAs play a supervisory role, it is the RBTs who directly engage with clients, implementing therapeutic interventions aimed at addressing behavioral challenges. This collaborative dynamic ensures a comprehensive approach to client care, with BCBAs providing guidance and RBTs executing tailored treatment plans.

ABA therapy serves as a cornerstone in the treatment of various conditions, most notably autism spectrum disorder and related developmental disorders. Its fundamental goal is to decipher the underlying causes of maladaptive behaviors and equip clients with the skills needed to navigate social interactions and daily challenges successfully. Through structured interventions and reinforcement techniques, RBTs facilitate meaningful progress in clients' ability to communicate, socialize, and engage in activities of daily living.

Central to the efficacy of ABA therapy is the RBT's ability to establish rapport and trust with clients, fostering a supportive environment conducive to learning and growth. RBTs undergo rigorous training to develop proficiency in implementing behavior management strategies, crisis intervention techniques, and data collection methods. Moreover, they continually refine their skills under the guidance of experienced BCBAs, ensuring adherence to best practices and ethical standards.

The significance of the RBT exam cannot be overstated, as it serves as a pivotal milestone in ensuring the competency and proficiency of individuals entering the field of ABA therapy. Beyond theoretical knowledge, the exam assesses practical skills, critical thinking abilities, and ethical decision-making, equipping RBTs with the tools necessary to navigate complex clinical scenarios.

In addition to working with individuals on the autism spectrum, RBTs encounter diverse populations with unique needs and challenges. From children with developmental delays to adults grappling with behavioral disorders, RBTs play a vital role in promoting independence, autonomy, and quality of life. Their interventions extend beyond the clinical setting, encompassing home-based services, school support, and community outreach initiatives.

As the demand for ABA therapy continues to grow, so too does the need for skilled and compassionate RBTs. The profession's ongoing evolution underscores the importance of continuous education and professional development, ensuring that RBTs remain at the forefront of evidence-based practice. By upholding standards of excellence and innovation, RBTs contribute to the ongoing advancement of behavioral healthcare and the well-being of those they serve.

The requirements for obtaining RBT certification reflect a commitment to excellence, professionalism, and ethical practice within the field of behavior analysis. By adhering to stringent standards and procedural protocols, the certification process ensures that RBTs are equipped with the knowledge, skills, and ethical framework necessary to make meaningful contributions to the lives of individuals receiving ABA therapy services.

Presently, a solitary Board Certified Behavior Analyst (BCBA) oversees the endeavors of numerous therapists, marking a pivotal aspect of the organizational structure within the realm of Applied Behavior Analysis (ABA) therapy. Delving into the prerequisites for aspiring therapists to embark on the journey toward becoming Registered Behavior Technicians (RBTs) reveals a multifaceted landscape of qualifications and procedural steps aimed at ensuring the highest standards of professionalism and competence in the field. Let's explore these requirements in detail:

- **Minimum Age Requirement and Career Preparation**: Prospective therapists must attain the age of 18 or older to qualify for RBT certification. This stipulation underscores the importance of early career exploration and preparation, prompting students to contemplate the pursuit of a career in ABA therapy as early as possible, ideally during their formative years in high school. Early exposure to the principles and practices of behavior analysis can foster a deeper understanding of the field and better equip individuals for the challenges and responsibilities inherent in therapeutic practice.

- **Comprehensive Background Check**: A crucial aspect of the RBT certification process is the completion of a comprehensive background check. This vetting procedure encompasses various facets, including a soft inquiry into the applicant's credit history. Analogous to background checks conducted within the purview of healthcare professions and educational settings, this scrutiny ensures the suitability and integrity of prospective therapists entrusted with the well-being and care of vulnerable populations. By upholding rigorous standards of integrity and professionalism, the field of behavior analysis endeavors to safeguard the interests and welfare of clients and maintain public trust and confidence.

- **Completion of a 40-Hour Training Course**: A cornerstone of the RBT certification process is the successful completion of a 40-hour training course, designed to impart essential knowledge and skills fundamental to the practice of behavior analysis. This comprehensive training regimen covers a diverse array of topics, ranging from behavioral principles and intervention techniques to ethical considerations and professional standards. Throughout the course, applicants are required to submit pertinent documentation pertinent to their certification candidacy, facilitating the evaluation process and ensuring compliance with certification requirements. Upon satisfactory completion of the training course, applicants receive notification regarding their eligibility to proceed with the RBT exam, marking a crucial milestone in their journey toward professional certification.

- **Proficiency Test**: Central to the certification process is the assessment of applicants' competency through a rigorous proficiency test. This evaluative measure serves as a litmus test of applicants' theoretical knowledge, practical skills, and ethical acumen, validating their readiness for clinical practice as Registered Behavior Technicians. By assessing candidates' understanding of core concepts in behavior analysis, their ability to apply evidence-based interventions, and their adherence to ethical guidelines, the proficiency test ensures that certified RBTs possess the requisite competencies to deliver effective, ethical, and culturally responsive care to diverse populations.

The journey toward RBT certification represents the initial step in a lifelong odyssey of professional growth, learning, and service. By embracing a commitment to continued education, mentorship, ethical practice, and credentialing, RBTs embody the ethos of excellence and dedication within the field of behavior analysis, ultimately enhancing the quality of care and outcomes for individuals receiving ABA therapy services.

Upon successful completion of the outlined prerequisites, aspiring RBTs must navigate the final hurdle: passing the RBT exam. Upon conquering this milestone, candidates unlock the gateway to embark on their professional journey within the realm of Registered Behavior Technicians. However, the culmination of the certification process merely marks the commencement of an ongoing commitment to professional growth and development.

- **Continued Professional Development**: While achieving RBT certification is a significant accomplishment, the quest for further knowledge and skill enhancement remains perpetual. Many therapists opt to pursue additional certifications throughout their careers, recognizing the invaluable benefits of lifelong learning and specialization. By continuously expanding their expertise through advanced certifications and specialized training programs, therapists fortify their proficiency and efficacy in delivering evidence-based interventions and addressing the diverse needs of their clientele.

- **Supervisory Oversight and Mentorship**: To maintain relevance and efficacy within the ever-evolving landscape of behavior analysis, RBTs must undergo supervised practice under the guidance of a Board Certified Behavior Analyst (BCBA). This supervisory arrangement not only ensures adherence to best practices and ethical standards but also fosters a culture of mentorship and professional collaboration. By leveraging the expertise and guidance of experienced BCBAs, RBTs gain invaluable insights and support, facilitating their growth and development as competent and compassionate practitioners.

- **Adherence to Ethical Standards**: Upholding strict codes of ethics is a cornerstone of professional practice within the field of behavior analysis. RBTs are obligated to adhere to the ethical guidelines prescribed by the certification board, ensuring the highest standards of integrity, confidentiality, and professionalism in their interactions with clients, colleagues, and stakeholders. By embodying ethical principles in their daily practice, RBTs uphold the trust and confidence of those they serve, fostering a culture of accountability and ethical responsibility within the profession.

- **Annual Certification Renewal**: The pursuit of excellence within the field of behavior analysis necessitates a commitment to ongoing credentialing and professional renewal. RBTs are required to renew their certifications annually, demonstrating their commitment to staying abreast of current research, best practices, and ethical guidelines. This annual renewal process serves as a mechanism for ensuring the currency and relevance of RBTs' knowledge and skills, thereby safeguarding the quality and integrity of behavior analysis services provided to clients.

MORE INFO ABOUT RBT EXAM

RBT certification represents not merely a professional accolade, but a testament to the dedication, resilience, and unwavering commitment to excellence epitomized by Registered Behavior Technicians. By embracing a proactive approach to preparation, harnessing collaborative learning opportunities, and demonstrating a thorough understanding of requisite competencies, aspiring RBTs embark on their certification journey equipped with the confidence and conviction to effect transformative change in the lives of individuals undergoing ABA therapy services.

Exploring the intricacies of RBT certification reveals its widespread acceptance and profound importance among the community of Board Certified Behavior Analysts (BCBAs) nationwide. This coveted certification serves as a beacon of professional competence and proficiency, assuring clinics, organizations, and parents that therapists possess the essential skills and knowledge to proficiently administer Applied Behavior Analysis (ABA) therapy under the watchful guidance of their clinical overseers.

At the heart of the RBT certification process lies a comprehensive 40-hour training course, serving as the bedrock of preparation for the ensuing examination. Within this immersive educational journey, prospective therapists are introduced to the foundational principles, methodologies, and ethical considerations intrinsic to behavior analysis. While this course provides a vital educational scaffold, candidates are encouraged to approach their preparation with proactive vigor and initiative, supplementing their learning with additional study aids and resources to deepen their grasp of critical concepts.

As the exam date draws near, diligent review and consolidation of course materials become paramount. Candidates are urged to immerse themselves in the study of pertinent course content, bolstered by the completion of practice questions and the creation of personalized study tools such as mnemonic devices or flashcards. Collaborative study sessions with peers or fellow course participants offer invaluable opportunities for reinforcement and knowledge exchange, fostering a supportive learning milieu conducive to success.

A comprehensive understanding of the RBT task list, comprising a diverse array of essential competencies and skills, is indispensable for exam readiness. By meticulously mastering each item on the task list and seeking clarification or additional guidance as necessary, candidates can fortify their confidence and preparedness, maximizing their chances of achieving success on the exam upon their initial attempt.

HOW TO PREPARE FOR THE RBT EXAM

Below are some recommendations to help applicants prepare for the RBT exam:

Ensuring Adequate Study Time:

It is imperative for prospective RBTs to allocate dedicated study periods to adequately prepare for the exam. This involves setting aside specific blocks of time in their schedules solely dedicated to reviewing course materials, practice questions, and supplementary resources essential for comprehensive exam readiness. By prioritizing study sessions and establishing a structured study routine, applicants can effectively manage their time and optimize their preparation efforts leading up to the exam date. Additionally, incorporating varied study techniques, such as active recall, concept mapping, and spaced repetition, can enhance retention and reinforce understanding of key concepts, thereby maximizing the efficacy of study sessions.

Minimizing Distractions by Creating an Optimal Study Environment:

It is essential for RBT exam candidates to cultivate a conducive study environment devoid of distractions. This entails identifying and mitigating potential sources of interruption to facilitate focused and effective study sessions. While background music can aid concentration for some individuals, it is advisable to exercise moderation and select music conducive to concentration. However, if music proves to be overly distracting, opting to study in silence may be beneficial. Additionally, candidates should proactively address potential distractions such as notifications from electronic devices, ambient noise, or interruptions from external sources. By curating a tranquil and distraction-free study space, candidates can optimize their cognitive engagement and enhance their ability to absorb and retain study materials effectively.

Focusing on Relevant Information:

Central to exam success is a comprehensive understanding of the RBT task list, a cornerstone of the examination. Prospective RBTs must prioritize thorough mastery of each component of this list, recognizing its pivotal role in determining exam performance. This involves meticulously studying and internalizing the specific tasks and competencies outlined in the RBT task list, ensuring fluency and proficiency in their application. Candidates should dedicate ample time to review and consolidate their knowledge of each task area, employing various study strategies such as concept mapping, mnemonic devices, and practice scenarios to reinforce comprehension and retention. By prioritizing the study of relevant information aligned with the RBT task list, candidates can bolster their readiness and confidence to navigate exam questions effectively and demonstrate mastery of essential competencies.

Enhancing Information Retention:

To optimize retention of necessary information, RBT exam candidates should employ a variety of effective study tools and techniques tailored to their individual learning preferences. Flashcards, for instance, offer a concise and portable means of reviewing key concepts and terminology, facilitating active recall and reinforcement of foundational knowledge. Similarly, engaging in mini-quizzes or self-assessment activities allows candidates to gauge their understanding of difficult areas and identify areas for further review. Additionally, completing individual practice tests under simulated exam conditions provides valuable opportunities to familiarize oneself with the exam format, refine time management skills, and pinpoint areas of strength and weakness. By incorporating these diverse study tools into their preparation regimen, candidates can enhance their ability to retain and recall necessary information crucial for success on the RBT exam.

Sustaining Motivation - Maintaining Focus on Goals and Benefits:

It is essential for RBT exam candidates to cultivate and sustain motivation throughout their preparation journey. One effective strategy is to establish a clear vision or mental image of the immediate benefits and long-term rewards associated with passing the exam. By visualizing the positive outcomes, such as career advancement opportunities, professional fulfillment, and the ability to make a meaningful impact in the lives of clients, candidates can harness intrinsic motivation to propel their study efforts forward. Additionally, setting specific, achievable goals and milestones can provide a sense of direction and purpose, helping candidates stay focused and committed to their preparation regimen. Moreover, cultivating a supportive network of peers, mentors, or study partners can offer encouragement, accountability, and perspective, fostering a sense of camaraderie and shared purpose. By nurturing a positive mindset, maintaining focus on their goals, and celebrating progress along the way, candidates can sustain motivation and momentum, ultimately increasing their likelihood of success on the RBT exam.

Prioritizing Rest and Recovery - Recognizing the Importance of Adequate Sleep:

While diligent studying is an integral aspect of exam preparation, it is equally crucial for RBT exam candidates to prioritize adequate rest and sleep. Without sufficient restorative sleep, candidates may enter the exam feeling fatigued and cognitively impaired, hindering their ability to focus, retain information, and effectively respond to exam questions. Therefore, it is imperative for candidates to establish a balanced study schedule that incorporates dedicated periods of rest and relaxation. This includes adhering to consistent sleep patterns, creating a conducive sleep environment, and implementing relaxation techniques to promote restful sleep. By prioritizing rest and recovery alongside their study efforts, candidates can optimize their cognitive functioning, enhance their concentration, and approach the exam with clarity, alertness, and readiness to perform at their best.

IS IT POSSIBLE TO RETAKE THE RBT EXAM?

Indeed, candidates are permitted to retake the RBT exam multiple times, with flexibility afforded for further attempts. However, there are certain parameters to consider within the framework of the certification process.

- **Retake Limitations**: While there is no restriction on the number of times one can retake the RBT exam, candidates are bound by a cap of eight attempts within each one-year authorization period. This regulatory measure aims to ensure that candidates maintain progress towards certification while allowing for reasonable opportunities for reevaluation and improvement.

- **First Attempt**: Should a candidate not succeed in passing the RBT exam on their initial endeavor, they are entitled to pursue subsequent retakes. It's noteworthy that approximately 50% of candidates who opt for a retake successfully pass the exam on their subsequent attempt. Therefore, diligent preparation and focused study are paramount for achieving success in the retake examination.

- **Managing Retakes**: In the event that a candidate exhausts their allotted eight attempts without achieving a passing score, but there remains time within their 12-month authorization period, they must adhere to a waiting period until the conclusion of the authorization period. Upon completion of the one-year timeframe, candidates may then proceed to reapply for certification and subsequently retake the exam, should they choose to pursue certification anew.

Navigating the process of retaking the RBT exam necessitates careful consideration of individual readiness, preparation strategies, and timelines. Candidates are encouraged to leverage resources such as study materials, practice exams, and mentorship opportunities to enhance their chances of success in subsequent attempts.

Additionally, maintaining open communication with supervising BCBAs and seeking guidance from experienced professionals can offer invaluable support and guidance throughout the certification journey. Ultimately, perseverance, resilience, and a commitment to continuous improvement are essential attributes for candidates embarking on the path towards RBT certification.

RETAKING THE RBT EXAM

Navigating the process of retaking the RBT exam involves several procedural steps to ensure a smooth and organized experience. By following the outlined procedures and considerations below, candidates can navigate the process of retaking the RBT exam with clarity, confidence, and readiness to achieve success on their subsequent attempt.

Here are the steps involved in the process of retaking the RBT exam:

1. **Accessing the Examination Retake Application:** Upon receiving notification of an unsuccessful exam attempt, candidates should promptly log into their online BACB (Behavior Analyst Certification Board) account. Within a window of 48 hours following the failed exam, candidates will discover an Examination Retake Application available for completion. This online form serves as the initial step in initiating the process of scheduling a retake exam.

Additional Details and Considerations:

- Candidates should ensure they have a stable internet connection and access to their BACB account credentials to facilitate the timely submission of the retake application.
- It's advisable for candidates to review any feedback or performance insights provided from their previous exam attempt to identify areas for improvement and inform their study strategies for the retake.

2. **Await Issuance of New Examination Authorization:** Upon submission of the Examination Retake Application, candidates can anticipate receiving a new examination authorization within 48 hours. This authorization serves as confirmation of eligibility to schedule and undertake the retake exam.

Additional Details and Considerations:

- Candidates should regularly monitor their email inbox and BACB account notifications to ensure timely receipt of the new examination authorization.
- It's essential to review any accompanying instructions or guidelines provided with the examination authorization to facilitate a seamless scheduling process.

3. **Adhere to Waiting Period Between Exam Attempts:** Candidates are required to observe a mandatory waiting period of at least seven days between successive exam attempts. This waiting period is designed to allow candidates adequate time for

reflection, review, and additional preparation before undertaking the retake exam.

Additional Details and Considerations:

- Utilize the waiting period effectively by engaging in targeted review of challenging topics, practicing sample questions, and implementing strategies to address areas of weakness identified from the previous exam attempt.
- Candidates may benefit from seeking guidance from mentors, study groups, or online resources to enhance their preparation efforts during the waiting period.

WHAT THE EXAM MEASURES

The administration of the RBT exam is overseen by a reputable testing company, which ensures the integrity and security of the examination process. This company hosts the exam on various websites, providing candidates with convenient access to the assessment while maintaining strict protocols to safeguard their personal information. Candidates can approach the exam with confidence, knowing that their data is protected and will not be shared with third parties.

As an online computer-based test, the format of the RBT exam aligns with standard academic assessments conducted via web platforms. This familiar format allows candidates to navigate through the exam with ease, focusing on demonstrating their competency in Applied Behavior Analysis (ABA). The exam evaluates candidates' proficiency across six task lists meticulously developed by the Behavior Analyst Certification Board (BACB).

Below are the six lists developed by the BACB:

1. Measurement:

When we talk about measurement in the context of the RBT exam, we're referring to the process of gathering important information during therapy sessions. This information helps therapists understand how behaviors change over time and whether the interventions they're using are effective. To do this, therapists use tools like graphs and data sets, which allow them to visually represent behavior patterns. By analyzing these patterns, therapists can identify trends and make informed decisions about the best course of action for their clients. In the context of autism therapy, measurement is particularly crucial because it helps therapists track progress and tailor interventions to meet each individual's unique needs.

2. Assessment:

In the context of the RBT exam, assessment refers to the process of understanding individual preferences. This means figuring out what each person likes or enjoys, which can vary from one individual to another. Therapists use various tools or methods to gather this information. For example, they might ask the person directly, observe their reactions to different options, or use structured assessments. Understanding preferences is important because it helps therapists tailor their interventions to better meet the needs and interests of each individual. This can make therapy sessions more engaging and effective.

3. Skill Acquisition:

In the RBT exam, skill acquisition refers to how therapists help clients learn new skills. ABA technicians, or therapists, need to understand the basics of creating plans to teach these skills. They have to figure out what each client needs to learn and break down the steps to help them achieve these goals. This process involves identifying the specific skills that are important for each client's development and designing structured plans to teach them effectively. By focusing on skill acquisition, therapists can support their clients in reaching their full potential.

In the field of Applied Behavior Analysis (ABA), skill acquisition is a fundamental aspect of therapy. It involves the systematic process of teaching individuals new skills or behaviors that are essential for their development and daily functioning. ABA technicians, also known as therapists or behavior technicians, play a critical role in facilitating skill acquisition for their clients, particularly those with autism spectrum disorder (ASD) or related developmental disabilities.

To effectively address the diverse needs of their clients, ABA technicians must possess a deep understanding of the principles and techniques underlying skill acquisition. This includes knowledge of behavior analysis principles such as reinforcement, shaping, prompting, and fading, which are instrumental in designing effective teaching strategies.

Moreover, ABA technicians are tasked with tailoring skill acquisition plans to meet the unique needs and preferences of each client. This involves conducting thorough assessments to identify areas of strength and areas requiring improvement, as well as determining the specific skills that are relevant and meaningful for the individual's overall development and quality of life.

Once the target skills have been identified, ABA technicians utilize evidence-based teaching strategies to systematically teach and reinforce these skills. This may involve breaking down complex skills into smaller, more manageable steps, providing clear and consistent instructions, modeling desired behaviors, and delivering positive reinforcement for successful attempts.

Throughout the skill acquisition process, ABA technicians continuously monitor their clients' progress and make necessary adjustments to the teaching strategies based on ongoing assessment data. This iterative approach allows therapists to individualize instruction, address any challenges or barriers that may arise, and maximize the effectiveness of the intervention.

By focusing on skill acquisition, ABA technicians empower their clients to acquire essential life skills, improve their independence and quality of life, and achieve their full potential. Moreover, by fostering a supportive and collaborative therapeutic environment, therapists facilitate meaningful learning experiences that promote engagement, motivation, and progress toward long-term goals.

4. Behavior Reduction:

Behavior reduction is about understanding why people behave in certain ways and how to help them change those behaviors if they're harmful or unwanted. Therapists look at the reasons behind a person's behavior, like whether it's to get attention or avoid something unpleasant. Then, they create plans to teach the person new, more positive ways of behaving. These plans, called interventions, are designed to address the root causes of the behavior and help the person learn healthier ways of coping and interacting with their environment.

In the context of Applied Behavior Analysis (ABA) therapy, behavior reduction focuses on understanding the underlying functions or reasons behind individuals' behaviors and implementing interventions to address problematic or challenging behaviors effectively.

Therapists begin by conducting a thorough assessment to analyze the function of the behavior, which involves identifying the specific triggers or antecedents that precede the behavior, as well as the consequences that follow. This functional analysis helps therapists understand why the behavior occurs and what purpose it serves for the individual.

Common functions of behavior in ABA therapy include seeking attention, escaping or avoiding a task or situation, obtaining access to desired items or activities, and self-stimulation or sensory seeking. By identifying the function of the behavior, therapists can develop targeted interventions to address the underlying causes and teach more adaptive or socially appropriate alternatives.

Interventions for behavior reduction are individualized based on the unique needs and characteristics of each client. Therapists may utilize a variety of evidence-based strategies, such as differential reinforcement, extinction, functional communication training, and antecedent-based interventions, to effectively reduce problematic behaviors and promote positive alternatives.

Moreover, therapists collaborate closely with clients, caregivers, and other members of the treatment team to develop comprehensive behavior intervention plans (BIPs). These plans outline specific strategies and techniques for addressing target behaviors, setting clear goals for behavior reduction, and monitoring progress over time.

Throughout the intervention process, therapists continuously assess the effectiveness of their interventions and make adjustments as needed based on ongoing data analysis and feedback. By providing consistent and structured support, therapists help individuals learn more adaptive ways of coping with challenges, improving their overall quality of life and social functioning.

5. Reporting and Documentation:

Reporting and documentation in ABA therapy require clear communication, efficient access to medical information, and adherence to legal and ethical standards to promote the well-being and progress of clients while maintaining professionalism and integrity in practice.

In ABA therapy, reporting and documentation involve two main aspects: communication with supervisors and adherence to legal and ethical guidelines.

- **Communication with Supervisors:** ABA technicians must effectively communicate with their supervisors regarding client progress, concerns, and any necessary updates. This includes providing regular updates on therapy sessions, discussing any challenges or successes, and seeking guidance or feedback when needed. Clear and timely communication with supervisors helps ensure that clients receive the best possible care and support.

- **Finding Medical Suggestions Quickly:** ABA technicians may need to access medical information or recommendations related to their clients' care. This could involve quickly locating relevant medical resources or consulting with healthcare professionals as needed to inform treatment decisions. Being able to efficiently find and utilize medical suggestions is essential for providing comprehensive and effective therapy services.

- **Understanding Legal and Ethical Guidelines:** ABA technicians are expected to have a solid understanding of the laws and guidelines that govern their practice. This includes knowledge of confidentiality laws, informed consent procedures, and professional codes of conduct. By adhering to legal and ethical guidelines, therapists ensure that they provide therapy services in a safe, ethical, and legally compliant manner.

6. Scope of Practice and Conduct:

In the field of ABA therapy, the scope of practice and conduct refers to the professional responsibilities and expectations that Registered Behavior Technicians (RBTs) must adhere to in their work. The scope of practice and conduct for RBTs emphasizes the importance of professionalism, interpersonal skills, and responsiveness in delivering effective ABA therapy services. By upholding these standards, RBTs can contribute to positive outcomes for their clients and maintain the integrity of the profession.

- **Building Relationships:** RBTs are required to establish positive relationships with colleagues, supervisors, and clients. This involves fostering a supportive and collaborative environment where open communication and mutual respect are valued. By building strong relationships, RBTs can effectively work as part of a team and provide high-quality care to their clients.

- **Responding to Feedback:** When feedback is provided, whether from supervisors, colleagues, or clients, RBTs should promptly acknowledge and respond to it. This includes actively listening to feedback, reflecting on areas for improvement, and implementing any suggested changes or recommendations. By being responsive to feedback, RBTs demonstrate a commitment to continuous learning and professional growth.

During the exam, candidates encounter more than 80 multiple-choice questions, of which over 70 contribute to their final score. Some questions are not included in the scoring process. Candidates have a total of one hour and 30 minutes to complete the exam.

PREPARING FOR EXAM DAY

As the day of the exam approaches, future therapists should plan to wake up early, ideally setting their alarms at least 30 minutes prior to the scheduled exam time. This allows ample time for last-minute preparations and ensures a stress-free arrival at the testing center.

On the day of the exam, testers must bring valid identification, preferably two forms, to verify their identity during the check-in process. This step is essential to facilitate a smooth registration process and avoid any delays or complications.

Personal belongings such as backpacks, books, and mobile phones are strictly prohibited in the testing area. Testers should plan to store these items in designated lockers or storage areas provided by the testing center to comply with security regulations and maintain the integrity of the examination environment.

Additionally, testers are advised not to bring food or beverages into the testing area. It's recommended to consume any necessary refreshments before the exam to avoid distractions and ensure that focus remains solely on the task at hand.

The exam itself is administered on a computer, with each test featuring a randomized set of questions categorized into identical topics. This randomized format minimizes the risk of cheating by preventing candidates from accessing pre-determined question sets. Moreover, the exam undergoes regular updates to ensure the relevance and accuracy of the content.

During the exam, it's crucial for testers to carefully read and understand each question presented. However, it's also important to manage time effectively and avoid spending too much time on any single question. Time management skills are essential to ensure that testers have sufficient time to answer all questions thoroughly without feeling rushed or pressured.

By following these guidelines and adequately preparing for exam day, future therapists can approach the RBT exam with confidence and maximize their chances of success.

SCORING PROCESS OF THE RBT EXAM

Upon completion of the RBT exam, testers promptly receive a notification indicating whether they have passed or not. Successful candidates who achieve a passing grade will receive their certification via email shortly after completing the exam. Typically, this email notification is sent out within a week, allowing testers to commence their job applications as Registered Behavior Technicians (RBTs) once they receive their certification.

In the event that a candidate does not pass the exam on their first attempt, they have the option to request a retake. Since the final quarter of 2020, the Behavior Analyst Certification Board (BACB) has implemented a policy allowing RBT applicants to retake the exam up to eight times within a one-year period, with minimal waiting periods between retakes, typically about a week or even less. Applicants do not need to reapply for the exam; instead, they receive an email containing instructions for scheduling their retake, including details on the time and location of the exam.

Moreover, the email may also provide valuable insights into the areas of the exam where applicants encountered the most difficulty. This feedback enables candidates to identify specific areas that may require additional attention and focus during their exam preparation, thereby enhancing their chances of success in subsequent attempts.

While the majority of applicants pass the exam on their first attempt, it's not uncommon for some individuals to require multiple attempts to achieve a passing score. Statistics indicate that approximately half of the applicants who initially fail the exam successfully pass on their second attempt, highlighting the importance of persistence and continued effort in pursuing RBT certification.

Overall, the scoring process of the RBT exam is designed to ensure that candidates demonstrate competence in the principles and practices of applied behavior analysis. Through multiple opportunities for retakes and valuable feedback, the BACB aims to support candidates in their journey toward becoming certified RBTs, ultimately contributing to the quality and professionalism of behavior therapy services.

www.ingramcontent.com/pod-product-compliance
Lightning Source LLC
Chambersburg PA
CBHW072258310526
45795CB00012B/1843